3 Silent Killers

3 Silent Killers:

Diabetes, Hypertension, Obesity

A Plain-Language Guide to a Healthier Lifestyle

Bob Hegamin

Edited by David K. Moody

All inquiries should be addressed to the editor:
David K. Moody
14419 Greenwood Avenue North, Suite A-203
Seattle, WA 98133

ISBN: 1493709798
ISBN-13: 9781493709793
Library of Congress Control Number: 2013920579
CreateSpace Independent Publishing Platform
North Charleston, South Carolina

Note to the Reader

Modern medicine often leaves us little time to ask our doctors why, how, and what's next. Medical professionals, on the other hand, routinely find themselves with too little time per patient and too many patients. Changing the mechanics of the medical system won't happen overnight.

After establishing that a diet change and exercise are routinely prescribed for treating disparate medical problems such as obesity, hypertension, and diabetes among others, I decided to find out how the two regimens contribute to maintaining the health of the patient.

I found myself reading a great deal of technical material and general information on the two. My findings and observations are being presented in this book as references only and not a substitute for a doctor's examination and recommendations.

I hope the information can help you determine how to keep yourself as healthy as possible based on the same two recommended regimens—diet change and exercise. If you suspect your medical problem is beyond the scope of this book I urge you to seek competent medical help.

Bob

My editor and I have made every effort to include the names of all references used in the writing of this book. We cannot ensure the accuracy and information contained herein, and can assume no responsibility for errors, inaccuracies, omissions, or inconsistencies in quotations used. Any slights of people, places or organizations are purely unintentional.

My thanks to my family and friends who gave me the support I needed with a special thanks to David Moody without whom I could not have finished this book.

Dedication

This book is dedicated to the following people:

- Those who have lost the battle to at least one of these three silent killers

- Everyone who fights the daily struggle against these killers to live for tomorrow

- Anyone who can use this information to make the necessary changes in their lifestyle now to prevent diabetes, hypertension, and obesity from destroying their lives

- Those who work valiantly and tirelessly to help people who are afflicted with any or all of these three deadly diseases

Table of Contents

The White House
Office of the Press Secretary
November 1, 2011

Presidential Proclamation—National Diabetes Month, 2011

NATIONAL DIABETES MONTH, 2011

BY THE PRESIDENT OF THE UNITED STATES OF AMERICA

A PROCLAMATION

Though we have made substantial progress in combating diabetes, the number of Americans burdened by this disease continues to grow at a rapid pace. During National Diabetes Month, we commemorate the work of caregivers, researchers, medical professionals, and advocates who lead the fight against diabetes, and we recommit to educating ourselves and our communities about how we can manage, treat, and prevent this disease. Diabetes can have a devastating impact on the health and well-being of those it affects, and it remains an urgent threat to our public health. In addition to immediate health issues, people with diabetes are more likely to suffer from complications such as heart attacks, strokes, high blood pressure, or kidney failure.

Most often diagnosed in young people, Type 1 diabetes inhibits the body's ability to produce insulin and can be managed with insulin injections, diet, and exercise. Research suggests that, unlike Type 1 diabetes, it is possible to prevent or delay Type 2 diabetes. Yet, Type 2 diabetes accounts for 90 percent of diabetes cases in the United States, and it continues to grow more prevalent in adults and children alike. It is essential that all Americans take steps to assess and reduce their risk of developing Type 2 diabetes by adopting a healthy diet, exercising regularly, and consulting a medical professional about their individual needs and risk factors.

My Administration remains committed to advancing diabetes education, research, prevention, and treatment. The National Diabetes Education Program—a partnership between the National Institutes of Health, the Centers for Disease Control and Prevention, and more than 200 public and private organizations to improve outcomes for people living with diabetes—encourages early diagnosis to prevent or delay the onset of Type 2 diabetes. In addition, the National Diabetes Prevention Program serves as part of a coordinated national strategy to reduce the prevalence of Type 2 diabetes by encouraging healthy eating habits and offering group support for adults who are striving to lose weight and get physically active. The Affordable Care Act ensures that all Americans joining a new health plan can receive recommended preventive services, like diabetes screenings, with no out-of-pocket costs. And, by 2014, Americans will not be denied insurance coverage because they have diabetes or other pre-existing conditions.

The increase in Type 2 diabetes among our Nation's children is linked to the rise of childhood obesity. To end the epidemic of childhood obesity within a generation, First Lady Michelle Obama's Let's Move! initiative is inspiring children to be physically active and empowering parents and caregivers to make healthy choices for their families. By encouraging our sons and daughters to develop healthy habits today, we help ensure they have a brighter, healthier tomorrow.

During National Diabetes Month, we remember those we have lost to diabetes, and we stand with the millions of Americans who have been touched by its consequences. As a Nation, it is our task to reduce the incidence of this illness and offer care and support to those it affects. This month and throughout the year, let us continue to pursue a diabetes-free future for our children, our families, and all Americans.

NOW, THEREFORE, I, BARACK OBAMA, President of the United States of America, by virtue of the authority vested in me by the Constitution and the laws of the United States, do hereby proclaim November 2011 as National Diabetes Month. I call upon all Americans, school systems, government agencies, nonprofit organizations, health care providers, research institutions, and other interested groups to join in activities that raise diabetes awareness and help prevent, treat, and manage the disease.

IN WITNESS WHEREOF, I have hereunto set my hand this first day of November, in the year of our Lord two thousand eleven, and of the Independence of the United States of America the two hundred and thirty-sixth.

Barack Obama

Chapter One

Digestion

When animals, including humans, appeared on the face of the earth, they instinctively knew they had to eat to stay alive.

Unlike all of the other animals, however, humans had the advantage of being able to gather plants and fruits or hunt and fish for their meals. They realized they didn't have to go hungry because they could pretty well eat whatever foods they happened to chance on.

As they established communities, they also learned to farm; to plant and harvest grains, vegetables, and fruits; and to breed animals that added meat, milk, and eggs to the supply and variety of food they had at their disposal.

This gave humans the ability to prepare and eat whatever pleased them the most, still ignorant that just eating and filling their stomachs was only the beginning of a process which was the real reason they continued to stay alive.

The basic foods eaten then and what we continue to eat today are, of course, the same raw materials the human body needs to transform into the essential nutrients for survival, namely, proteins, fats, carbohydrates, vitamins, and minerals. While not considered a nutrient, water must be included because without it there would be no life on earth.

Even today, most people still believe that nourishing the body is the act of simply putting food in their mouths to fill their stomach.

They may know, or maybe not, that the process of digestion starts in the mouth, where an enzyme in the saliva reacts with whatever assortment of food has just been eaten. Without any conscious effort, the person's teeth will automatically grind and pulverize solids into pieces small enough to swallow and make the trip of the mix to the stomach easy and uneventful.

That part of the digestive process that started in the mouth stops when it reaches the stomach, where other enzymes take over. The new, still partly solid mix in the stomach, though, is not yet in a form that can be used by the trillions of cells in the human body.

The stomach, however, has been programmed to churn and blend the mix into a consistency which takes between one and four hours to empty into the small intestine, where even more enzymes are added. It eventually becomes a nutrient-laden liquid specifically formulated to pass through the intestinal walls and into the bloodstream for delivery to those trillions of cells.

Whether we realize or care what our digestive process is doing for us, there are a couple of factors in general about our daily diets that should concern us. First, in our youth we adopted marginal eating habits that have stuck with us through the years.

This brings us to our second point which is that many of us have continued the habit of eating poorly. One day we will suddenly discover that we've put on weight, and more distressingly, inches around our waist. But, better late than never, we look for ways to take corrective action.

Do we have to learn the hard way that our body doesn't process food the same way it did when we were younger? The day will come when we have to face reality. Two other factors have also been contributing to our increasing weight and growing girth. One is that we've been feeding our body the "wrong" kinds of food and the other is that we've aged.

As mature caring adults, is it too late to do anything about the situation now?

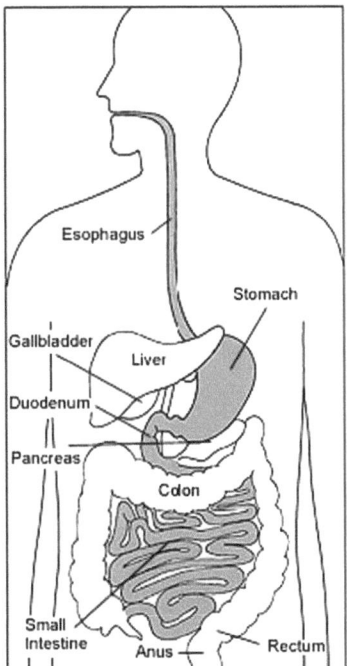

Image 1: Upper GI (upper gastrointestinal tract)

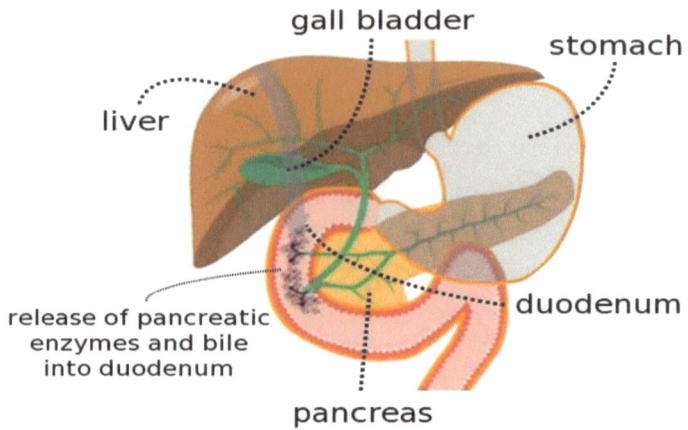

Image 2: Digestive System

Without realizing it, our metabolism--the amount of energy (calories) required for daily activities--decreases gradually. Simply stated, our bodies just don't need all the food we're eating. However, the changes have been subtle, so we had no reason to eat less. Consequently, the excess calories have been storing up as fat, which is the body's energy source in emergencies. In past centuries, catastrophes were common. In modern times, though, famine and such shortages are rare in most industrialized nations.

As a result, we've put on weight, and in all probability most of us have tried to solve the problem by buying into some "magic-bullet" diet plan or some exercise program. And, despite spending a great deal of time, effort, and money for some temporary weight loss, our pounds generally return with a vengeance anyway.

Chapter Two

Calories

Stop eating so much garbage!
Quit snacking and drinking all those sodas!

Those were words of wisdom years ago because "garbage" was any fattening food, while snacks and sodas were sources of so-called "empty" calories. But consider those words today now that we know a calorie is only a unit of heat or energy *produced* by food as it is burned to fuel the body's engine. That bears repeating: A calorie is just a unit of energy and not a food. If that's the case, how does it put weight on us? That's just the point, it doesn't.

Unfortunately, countless factoids about health and obesity have caused us to place an undue emphasis on the number of calories *inherent* in the foods we eat rather than on the amount or types. The technical reasons explaining the differences have always been available, but they're typically explained in language that is not easy to understand. They had shown time and again that health professionals are right: Diets full of fat and soda are not nutritious and do nothing to keep a person healthy. The information they have had available, however, has just not been up to the job of telling us why.

Being overweight or obese is the combination of both our diet and our advancing age. Over the years, our increasing weight and growing waistline had been telling us to put a stop to bad eating habits or at least change our lifestyle.

Because we've ignored the symptoms until now, this is a good time to say something about our growing waistline as a sign that two subversive and deadly diseases have been developing right along with it — Type 2 Diabetes and Hypertension (high blood pressure).

Losing excess weight today should be a primary goal not just for its own sake but because we will be facing some serious consequences if we don't. Did you know that there is a strong relationship between being overweight and hypertension? With that in mind, do you know what *your* blood pressure is? If not, you should check it regularly and often.

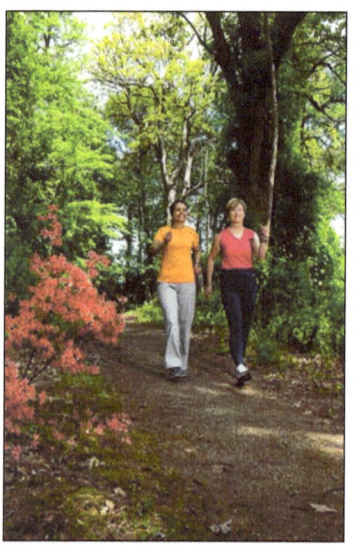

Image 3: Researchers found that at least 30 minutes a day of walking, jogging, or other weight-bearing activity, in addition to being heart healthy, is needed to maintain bone health.

If your numbers are consistently above "normal", you might have a hypertension problem. In fact, you most likely aren't going to be able to take care of it by yourself.

When the blood pressure machine gives you the results it's programmed to give, it has done its job. Indirectly, though, it's also telling you Type 2 diabetes might be in your future.

To better understand the relationship among obesity, hypertension, and Type 2 Diabetes and help overcome the threats of all three simultaneously, the simplest and least expensive things you can do to help yourself are to *eat less and exercise more*! You've heard that before—the common sense approach to all three problems that doctors and nutritionists have been advocating for years.

This calls for a *warning*: Getting examined and tested by your doctor is the only certain way to determine your exact medical condition. *DON'T GUESS*! What else can we do for ourselves when we don't know what our present diet is actually doing to or for us? If hypertension and diabetes are manifestations of being overweight, how is food contributing to their development?

First, let's try to understand what we're dealing with. Because being "fat" or obese is the only observable symptom that anything is wrong and may be harming us, let's start with the *"calorie"* in food and go from there.

Packaged foods are no-brainers! Their labels tell us how many calories each portion or serving will provide our body. It also tells us the package contains so many servings, such as five of 500 calories each. But have you noticed that the labels also include other information about ingredients such as fat, cholesterol, sodium, protein, carbohydrates, sugar and—if you're lucky—dietary fiber and potassium? While those ingredients are in your stomach, what do you think they're doing while their calories are being turned into energy the body needs to keep you alive?

Although they're necessary for our nutrition, they're also *competing* warriors in the battle over whether hypertension and Type 2 diabetes will become more of a problem, along with our waistline.

The implied warning from the label is this: If you eat more than the suggested single portion, in addition to other foods at any one sitting, you might be asking for more trouble than just putting on some weight.

Fresh fruits and vegetables don't have labels, don't contain very many calories, and are free of the additives that packaged foods contain. Just as nature intended, fruits and vegetables don't generally pose a problem. Their skin provides fiber, and their "meat" delivers natural sugars and carbohydrates.

Drinking juice is not as healthy as eating fruit. A typical glass of apple or orange juice can contain the sugar content of four or five pieces of fruit, yet none of the fiber and other nutrients. Fruit juice does not provide a balanced diet of fruit or vegetable servings. While some fruits and vegetables are intended to be peeled, nature has packaged most of them to be consumed as they exist in nature—with the skin on.

If a doctor has not advised you to stay away from specific foods, why not just fight the obesity problem by eating more fruits and vegetables and less of everything else?

Obviously, the first common-sense thing we can do to prevent putting on even more weight, let alone take it off, is to learn how and why we must cut some high-calorie foods out of our diets.

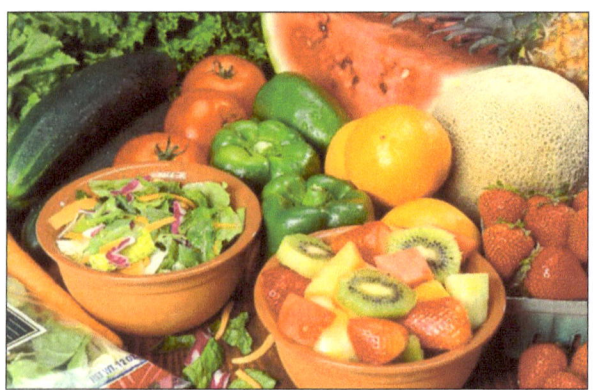

Image 4: Fruits and vegetables provide one of the best ways to satisfy your diet with what nature intended.

To start, let's first understand that foods we typically find on our grocery shelves fall into three general categories and contain everything necessary to keep us alive, fit, and healthy. The editors of *Eat and Heal* present these three categories as follows:

(1) Carbohydrates — Breads, cereals, fruits, and vegetables supply our body with carbohydrates—starches and sugars that are transformed into glucose which the internal organs as well as the rest of the body use as fuel for their daily activities.

(2) Proteins — Meats, fish, milk, beans, peas and grains provide us with the protein that is the main component in skin, muscles, bones, and most other body parts.

(3) Fats — Dairy products, eggs, meats, and oils contain fats that serve several purposes, including transportation of fat-soluble vitamins—A, B, E, and K—to cells, and storing energy"[1]

Because we know so much about what types of foods we should be eating, why are our diets still causing so many of our health problems?

Why ask? We already have the answer: we're eating too much and definitely much too much of the "wrong" kind.

More to the point, aren't we reminded constantly that we're consuming too much fat, especially too much of the saturated kind? Consequently, many commercials are designed to promote products that allegedly will keep our cholesterol numbers low. Others tell us to eat less and exercise more. Companies follow up by producing low-fat foods for the marketplace.

This leaves us with commercials that tell us we'll remain forever "regular," keep us healthy, and keep our stomachs feeling full longer if we use their products containing fiber. On a different level, still other commercials remind us to stay away from salt and sugar.

Gloria Rose, Director of the Gourmet Long Life Cooking Schools also cautions us with the following: "All foods we take in are converted at one time or another into sugar (aka glucose) because sugar is the unit of fuel that the cells of our body need. Sugar cannot get into most cells without insulin providing entry. An absolute deficiency of insulin or an insensitivity to insulin action leads to an elevated blood sugar."[2]

It looks like losing weight will be a never-ending fight because everything we eat eventually turns to sugar (a.k.a. glucose). But wait! Before all that can happen, insulin must be present.

All we need to know now is that cells need fuel to keep operating. Specifically, that fuel is glucose which to the body is as gasoline with additives is to our car's engine. All the food we eat goes into making the mixture that eventually becomes "glucose." The body's engine determines how much from each of the food categories it needs. So, let's look at the three food categories essential for our lives:

Carbohydrates   Protein   Fat

Chapter Three

Carbohydrates

Once humans started living as members of communities and developing societies, they began to prepare meals that kept them alive and healthy to do the jobs they set out to do. Many societies settled on diets around rice, and others found the potato more plentiful. Still others took the time and effort to grind wheat, turn it into flour, and prepare pasta and bread from it.

What each society had determined naturally was that the basic foods

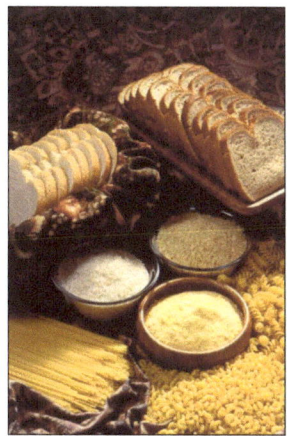 contributing to longevity of life were from plants growing around their towns and villages. As time went on, they cultivated and harvested crops of those same plants, which today we call plant carbohydrates. The authors of *The Glucose*

Image 5: Rice, pasta, cornmeal

Examples of complex carbohydrates

Revolution emphasize that development with the following: "In fact, carbohydrate is the most widely consumed nutrient in the world, after water. It's important to the human body because it yields glucose."[3]

Fortunately, over time we have learned even more about carbohydrates, including the fact that there are several types. This is important because we might find ourselves living in environments or societies that provide foods different from those we grew up with. If that were to happen, we would have to learn how to choose the "right" kinds of carbohydrates to sustain our normal lifestyle.

To help understand and select the "right" carbohydrates for our individual needs, the following are the only two considerations offered universally: *Simple* carbohydrates, called sugars, include the natural sugars found in milk, fruits, and vegetables as well as white table sugar and honey. *Complex* carbohydrates, called starches, include foods like rice, beans, potatoes, and pasta.[4]

But, before we go on, additional features about simple carbohydrates are that they are essentially one-or-two-molecule sugars, can enter the bloodstream rapidly, and cause a fast rise in blood glucose, accompanied by a rise in insulin.[5]

We've all witnessed children in organized sports served orange juice or a piece of orange during a break in their activities. What was given was a shot of instant energy thanks to simple carbohydrate sugar, but it was used up immediately in the rest of the game and didn't hang around to be stored as fat.

Once again, simple carbohydrates break down into glucose quickly and can be used immediately, but in doing so also cause a fast rise in blood glucose. We can conclude then that complex carbohydrates are processed into glucose at a slower rate, used more slowly which contributes to a slower rise in blood glucose.

Are simple and complex carbohydrates different in other ways? *Yes, they are.* As carbohydrates they're both organic compounds comprised of carbon, hydrogen and oxygen atoms. We know that the simple carbohydrate in its most basic form is just one sugar molecule. On the other hand, the complex carbohydrate is a long chain of simple carbohydrates or sugar molecules *chemically* linked together.

All of this bears repeating now because it's the key to understanding obesity, hypertension and diabetes. The critical difference between the simple and complex carbohydrate is that the simple carbohydrate is quickly turned into glucose and can be utilized almost immediately causing the *blood glucose level* to rise sharply. On the other hand, complex carbohydrates release their sugars more slowly. The questions are: Why are they slower and, secondly why is it so important to know?

I think we now know enough to be able to answer that question because many of you have been asking why and how our *blood glucose level* rises rapidly.

Let's focus on "fiber" first, which, if included in our meals, will keep our stomachs full longer—at least that's what TV commercials tell us!

Historically, people in the good old days were told that if they wanted to stay healthy their diets had to include "roughage' which meant eating an adequate supply of vegetables and cereals. Today we're more explicit knowing that vegetables and cereals are good for us if for nothing else than to keep us "regular" because of the fiber they contain. So, let's look at fiber.

Chapter Four

Fiber

One of the unique features of carbohydrate-rich plant foods is dietary fiber, which is the indigestible component of plant cell walls. The authors of *The Glucose Revolution* tell us: "There are two general types of fiber. *Insoluble fiber* is the "roughage" found in vegetables and the skins and outer coatings of grains, fruits, and legumes (peas and beans), while *soluble fiber,* so called because it dissolves or forms a gel-like substance when mixed in water. It is abundant in beans, oats, and fruits."[6]

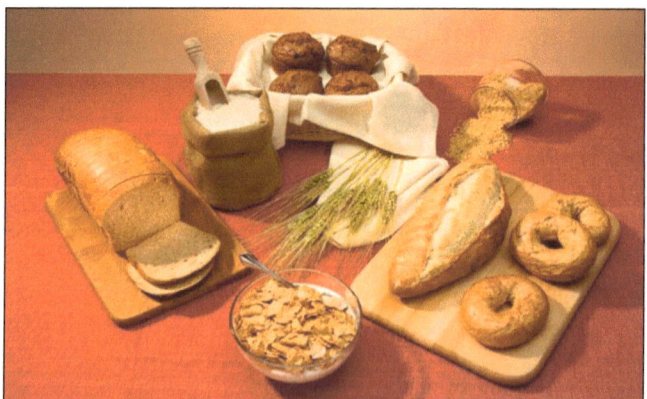

Image 6: Grain products with 2.5 grams or more of fiber per serving: bran muffins, brown rice, whole-wheat loaf bread, whole-wheat bagels, whole-grain cereal, whole-wheat sliced bread, and whole-wheat flour.

In Chapter 1, I said that once the food you've eaten reaches your stomach, enzymes take over. If you've also consumed foods that contain fiber, the partly solid mix will now take on a taffy-like consistency—thick and gooey—instead of remaining "watery." Not yet in a form the body's cells can use, the stomach continues to churn away at the mix no matter how gooey, and, when signaled that it's ready for the next step, dumps the mix into the small intestine. There, even more enzymes are added but later than normal because fiber had slowed down the process.

This will spread out the production of glucose over time and prevent a fast rise in insulin. On our own, what better way is there for us to help slow the production of glucose than by creating a series of delays? It will happen every time fiber is added to the diet because the food from the stomach is delayed getting to the intestine.

The plan is simple to implement. Just choose carbohydrates that are fibrous and hard to chew which means it will take an extraordinary amount of time to break down in the stomach. There is a universal daily recommendation of 25 to 35 grams of fiber to maintain good health, so wouldn't it be in our best interest to look for vegetables and prepared foods with lots of fiber?

It's going to take more time to empty the stomach than it normally would, which also means it will take longer to be hungry again. You've got to admit that it's certainly worth a try for so little effort.

Once again! We must slow down the digestive process by selecting more foods that contain fiber, which means eating more foods from the complex carbohydrate group.

This time the authors of *The Glucose Revolution* emphasize the following: "Viscous fiber thickens the viscosity or thickness of the mixture in the digestive tract. This slows the passage of food and restricts the movement of enzymes, thereby slowing digestion. The end result is a lower blood sugar response."[7]

Chapter five

Protein

By now you're probably saying: Wait a minute! Not all of us are vegetarians! It's true that not all of us are, but let's consider the issue from the standpoint that carbohydrates are generally inexpensive enough to allow most families to still enjoy nutritious and healthy meals.

In grocery stores, protein sections are typically labeled "Meat," "Poultry," "Fish," and "Dairy." You won't find cereals and legumes like peas, beans, and peanuts in those sections because they're carbohydrates. The body treats them like proteins though--a source of low-cost protein for your meals.

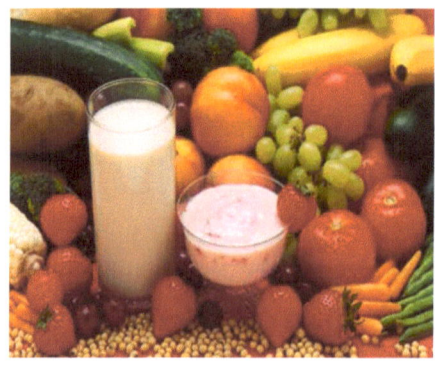

Image 7: A diet rich in cereals, legumes and other non-meat proteins add variety to your diet as well as being good for you.

The body knows what it needs to keep itself healthy so it processes whatever food we eat to meet those needs. Besides breaking carbohydrates down into glucose, our digestive juices have the additional jobs of breaking down incoming proteins and reforming them into what are called amino acids, which when bonded together form the human protein.

In his book titled *High Blood Pressure Relief Diet*, author James Scala says: "Visualize a protein as a long string of 22 different beads that can be linked together in any number of 3 or more with no upper limit."[8]

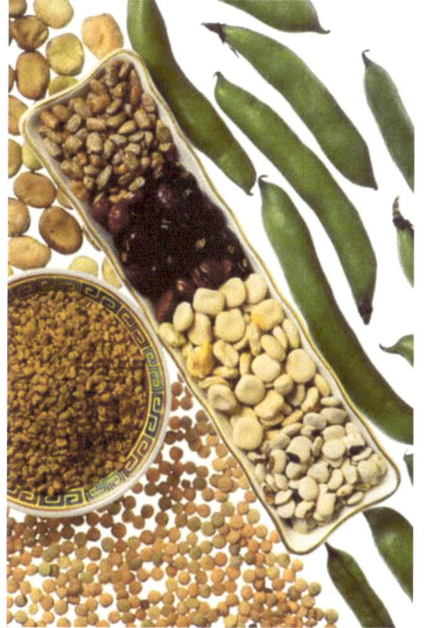

Image 8: Legumes provide a rich diversity of tastes and textures. This class of vegetable includes beans, peas, and lentils, and are among the most versatile and nutritious foods available. Legumes are typically low in fat, contain no cholesterol, and are high in minerals such as folate, iron, magnesium, and potassium. This versatile food group contains beneficial fats and soluble and insoluble fiber. Lower in fat and cholesterol, legumes can be a healthy protein source to substitute for meat.

Described as the building block of tissue, amino acids are used to maintain our organs and skeleton as well as our muscles, skin, and hair.

Although there are twenty-two known amino acids, the body can produce only thirteen on its own. Author Scala says, "The nine that we can't make are called 'essential' because without these, we cannot live. These essential amino acids must be provided by the protein we get from the food that we eat."[9]

You can do your part in supplying the other nine by eating protein-rich foods such as meat, eggs, fish, poultry, milk, cheese, cereals, peas, beans, and nuts. This is important because the body needs all 22 amino acids to remain healthy.

So remember this when preparing your daily diet! If you cannot get enough energy from carbohydrates, your body will start using protein from muscle mass to meet its needs. When the condition goes on too long, the body will begin losing muscle tone, which is a symptom that some muscles are wasting away.

Let's look at the situation from another perspective to make the point. The brain needs protein to survive so while you're asleep for the eight or ten hours between meals your brain has been using protein for fuel.

Because the body doesn't store amino acids or proteins as it does carbohydrates or fats, it needs a daily supply of amino acids to make new protein. So keep this in mind: The benefits of eating a handful of peanuts or almonds as a snack now and then outweigh the fact that they are **a** little high in calories.

Chapter Six

Fat

We like to think of ourselves as being just a little "fat" but our doctors look at us and see "obese." You ask: "How could that be?" but, doesn't this sound familiar? I just haven't eaten that much! All I had for breakfast this morning was a Danish and a cup of coffee. For lunch, I'm having a burger, fries and a shake. Tonight, we're joining a couple of friends for dinner at our favorite restaurant. Consciously, we haven't eaten that much fat.

Yet here we are complaining about our weight and the fact that our clothes aren't fitting our frame that well any more. It's obvious we're going to have to rethink how we put fat on ourselves to understand why our girth is expanding.

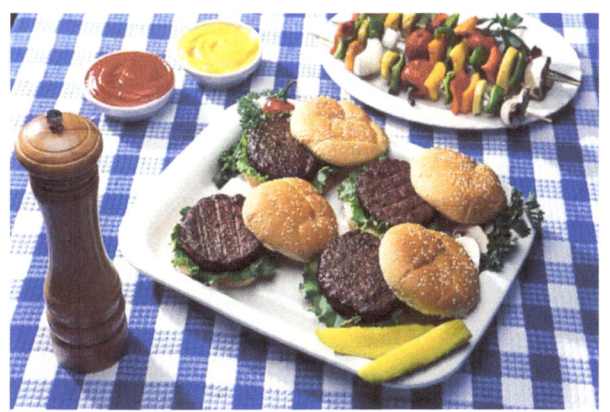

Image 9: While meat is a great source of protein, how it is prepared and served can make a healthy meal into one loaded with additional calories from fat, condiments, and sauces. Remember that moderation is key.

Like the other categories of food we've discussed so far, fat is a source of calories and nourishment the body needs to survive. But fat contains twice as many calories per gram weight as carbohydrates and protein.

Fitness expert and author Robert K. Cooper says, "Gaining new body fat from large doses of dietary fat can be amazingly easy (…) because your body dramatically increases the production of the hormone insulin when you gulp down high-fat foods (…) one of the effects of insulin is to increase your appetite and the rate at which your body stores fat."[10]

That explains why your will power keeps breaking down as you try to reduce. It seems that every time you eat some high-fat food, a surplus of insulin is being poured into your system, making certain your appetite increases even more.

We've all shopped enough to know that fat is inherent in the meat products we purchase. But we don't mind because we like the taste of cooked dietary fat in bacon, steaks, pork chops, chicken, etc., don't we?

However, you should realize that the "triglyceride" fat that makes up part of your chicken, pork, or steak meal actually creates a major problem. You can tell it's around when you see traces of grease on your plate and silverware. It's a substance made up of fat molecules which only a solvent can remove.

We've got a problem. Fat molecules are large—too large for the digestive enzyme in the stomach to process. They must get into the intestine. In other words, fats we just consumed can't be stored for fuel or used in the near future.So, how does the body deal with this problem?

Fortunately, the body has its own way of solving problems. In this case it emulsifies the molecules, that is, reduces their size with bile. Created in the liver, it's stored in the gallbladder until needed. When fats show up in the small intestine, the gallbladder excretes the bile.

In the intestine and together with another specialty enzyme from the pancreas, the bile eventually reduces all of the large globules of tri-glyceride fat we just ate into microscopically small water-soluble glob-ules. In this form, fat is allowed to pass through the intestinal wall and eventually ends up in the bloodstream.

Edwin Kiester, the author of *Eating Healthy Cookbook*, explains it this way: "A new kind of fat is produced within the (intestinal) wall and passes first into the lymphatic system and then into the bloodstream for processing by the liver and the muscles of the body and finally is stored in adipose tissue—what is commonly called fat."[11]

Something is going on here! In this chapter (endnote 10), we learned that the body will also produce "the hormone insulin when you gulp down high-fat foods." The question is: Why? This new supply of insulin isn't needed to open cell doors because fat is not glucose.

Instead, it just adds to the congestion in the arteries and contributes to obesity. As Dr. Cooper says, "When you eat high-fat foods, you'll prob-ably just want to eat more high-fat foods in the hours that follow."[12]

There's only one conclusion you can come away with from this dis-cussion: If you want to lose weight, you're going to have to cut down eat-ing high-fat foods for which the pancreas will be providing insulin the body doesn't need at this time.

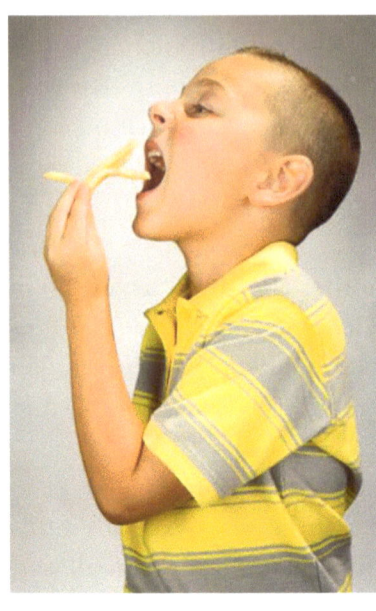

Once again, the moral of the story is: *Reduce your intake of high-fat foods.*

Image 10: French fries, loaded with fat and calories

When we start craving unhealthy snacks because they "taste good" we've put ourselves on the path of getting fat. Our body automatically reacts by storing the extra calories provided by such foods instead of using them for fuel.

But here's an interesting fact: Although fat carries twice the energy punch per gram than carbohydrates do some carbohydrates can produce a type of fat that could put a person with diabetes at a higher risk of heart disease:

In the *Doctor's Book of Food Remedies*, author Selene Yeager says, "(Some) carbohydrates still raise blood sugar faster than protein or fat do. This (…) can increase levels of triglycerides, a type of fat that has been linked with a higher risk of heart disease in people with diabetes."[13]

What are triglycerides? Buzzle.com author Shrinivas Kanade defines them this way: "Triglycerides, sometimes also referred to as 'ugly fats,' are fats that we derive from the diet and from carbohydrates in the body to fulfill our energy requirements."[14]

Let's look at this again because carbohydrates aren't supposed to do this to us. And they don't. At least the complex carbohydrates don't!

What actually happens is that when you take in more calories from simple carbohydrates than you need immediately, your body will eventually transform the excess into triglyceride fat in addition to those we normally consume in meats.

It seems that both fatty foods and simple carbohydrates can contribute to forming triglyceride fats. The moral of this section comes from livestrong.com, the website of The Livestrong Foundation: "Keep your triglyceride levels down by seeking complex carbs such as legumes, whole-grain foods, fruits, and vegetables; selecting lean meat such as fish and poultry; and consuming your fats as mostly unsaturated fats, such as those found in olive oil, nuts, seeds, and canola oil."[15]

We've talked about triglycerides and diabetics, but is triglyceride fat also a danger to those who don't have the disease? The answer is a definite *yes!*

To explain, let's go back to the article by Shrinivas Kanade who adds this: "The excess amount of these (triglycerides) can get deposited on the inner walls of the blood vessels and can lead to various kinds of heart disease and stroke."[16]

That's something we should all be thinking about! So, let's examine "fat" a little more. First, advertisers have already told us a great deal about saturated, polyunsaturated, and mono-unsaturated fats.

Obliquely, commercials have been emphasizing the fact that meat products with a great deal of saturated fat should be used very sparingly. As author Selene Yeager says, "Eating too much of any type of fat, including the relatively healthful monounsaturated fats is likely to cause weight gain, which is something that people with diabetes simply can't afford."[17]

At this point, you have to appreciate the additional explanation that follows since you already know that sugar, a.k.a. glucose brings out an immediate insulin response. You now also know that throughout your entire life you've been hit with this "no-brainer" which Dr. Cooper describes as follows: "The most potent fat-promoting foods seem to be those that are high in both fat and sugar, which describes some of America's most popular foods. Just think of cake, ice cream, doughnuts and chocolate candy—all ponderous mixtures of fat and sugar...the sugar in those foods stimulate the production of insulin at the same time that large amounts of fat are entering the bloodstream... readying the 'fat' cells for storage."[18]

That makes sense! As soon as the body senses glucose, insulin is excreted to unlock the cells. However, the fat hasn't been emulsified so it can't get into the cells with the glucose.

On this point, Selene Yeager says, "Consuming fewer carbohydrates and using more monounsaturated fats will lower triglyceride levels, as well as the dangerous fat-storing LPL enzyme. Good sources of monounsaturated fats include olive oil, avocados, and many nuts.[19]

We've just been introduced to LPL described as a dangerous fat-storing enzyme. That should concern us. But, *Why*? Just what is LPL, and why is it dangerous?

Here is how fitness expert Clarence Bass defines it: "LPL is an enzyme that hangs out on the walls of the tiny blood vessels in your fat tissue and in your muscles. It decides whether to extract the fat particles that pass by and store them in your fat cells or, alternatively, pass them into your muscles cells to be burned as energy."[20]

It seems we can make an assumption here because we're probably talking about previously emulsified fats in the bloodstream. The quote by Clarence Bass says that LPL can either store them directly into fat cells or put them in your muscles for fuel.

The assumption here is that glucose is also in the bloodstream at the same time. When the muscle cell door opens both fat and glucose will enter. Because glucose is primarily a fuel it will be consumed first. The remaining fat will remain in the cell and eventually become a part of a new fat cell.

Fat can come to us in different forms, such as *oils* used in cooking and in salads; *nuts* such as peanuts, cashews, and walnuts; *fish* such as salmon, tuna, and sardines; and *dairy products* such as milk, ice cream, cheese, and butter.

So, what does fat have to do with the onset of diabetes? Those with diabetes will tell you that for years they have been advised to keep their intake of fat to small quantities, and wisely, for two very important reasons, which were summarized in a fact sheet published by the International Diabetes Institute in 2003 as follows:

> **Weight control.** Excess body fat, particularly abdominal fat prevents *insulin* from working properly which leads to raised blood glucose levels. In addition, reducing fat intake, together with more physical activity, will help control weight and therefore help control blood glucose levels.

> **Heart disease risk.** People with diabetes are at greater risk of heart disease and circulation problems. Reducing fat, especially saturated fat, will help to reduce this risk.[21]

The Diabetes Fact sheet also helps put the issue of fat in the proper frame of reference. Although written relative to diabetes, it answers the basic question: If I don't consciously eat fat, where does it come from to become part of me?

> **Hidden Fats** Processed meats e.g. salami, bacon, nuts, avocado, olives, potato chips, and snack foods (…) cakes, biscuits, (sweet and dry)

pastries, croissants, chocolate, and fried and takeaway foods, pate, dips, milk, cheese, yogurt and ice cream.

Added Fats Butter, oil, margarine, cream, mayonnaise, and salad dressing[22]

From that perspective, we've got to look at fat as being an ingredient in many foods we eat. It's simply a matter of being aware that it's there and adjust our eating habits and diets accordingly.

Like carbohydrates and protein, there are some fats that are "good" and some "bad." To go on, it's a matter of determining which is which. As a generalization, foods that can produce a fat that hardens at room temperature are the seriously "bad" saturated fats and foods.

Consequently, you should avoid or only occasionally consume any type of food whose fat content exhibits such a characteristic.

With that in mind, many nutritionists recommend that when cooking at home you use olive and canola oils that are considered "good" fats.

So, when purchasing condiments such as mayonnaise and salad dressings read the label to see if they have also been prepared with at least one of the two recommended oils.

It's not to say that fats should not be used or consumed at all, but those mentioned in this article are provided to alert you to the fact that fats may already be used in foods you're eating in your daily diet without your knowing it. So, be ever diligent!

To make certain you get an adequate supply of "good" fat in your diet, consider fish such as salmon, tuna, and sardines and (surprisingly) some leafy green vegetables, which are all sources of omega 3.

The omega 3 fatty acid or simply "omega 3" refers to a polyunsaturated fatty acid that can remain liquid at room temperature or refrigerated.

It is essential for providing protection against heart disease and strokes with other possible benefits for cancer, lupus and rheumatoid arthritis.

The authors of *Eat and Heal* explain why fish oil is good for you: "Studies show the fish oil keeps your blood from sticking together, keeps your veins wide open, and helps your heart to beat regularly. Keeping your veins open and blood flowing easily is important in preventing heart attacks and strokes."[23]

Don't like fish? Then use flaxseed as a supplement. The George Mateljan Foundation explains why: "The warm, earthy, and subtly nutty flavor of flaxseeds combined with an abundance of omega-3 fatty acids makes them an increasingly popular addition to the diets of many a health-conscious consumer. Whole and ground flaxseeds, as well as flaxseed oil, are available throughout the year."[24]

Vegetarians might also consider using fish oil supplements as a substitute as well as flaxseed for any of the recommended cold water fish.

If none of the foods or substitutes will work for you, you can always eat some walnuts that are also high in omega 3 fats.

Chapter Seven

Insulin

I've gone through a lot of steps to explain how and why our weight and girth are increasing. However, I haven't said a word about how diabetes and hypertension, two of our three silent killers, were developing at the same time. Just as in daily life, we tend to get distracted by what is observable, more worried about our weight and growing waistline than we are about the other two life-threatening conditions that constantly face us.

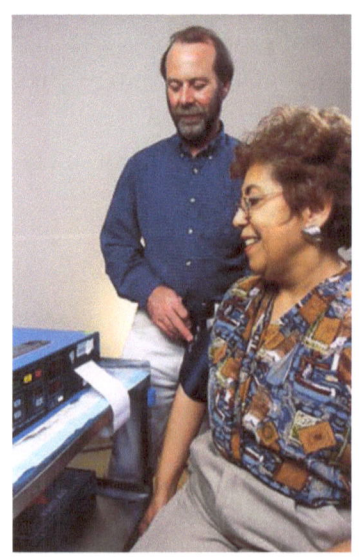

Image 11: An Endocrinologist checks a volunteer's blood pressure in a study of diets high in fructose or glucose. These sugars affect production of leptin and insulin, hormones that regulate appetite.

Consequently, a quote from Chapter 2 is worth repeating here: "All foods we take in are converted at one time or another into sugar (aka glucose) because sugar is the unit of fuel that the cells of our body need. Sugar cannot get into most cells without insulin providing entry. An absolute deficiency of insulin or an insensitivity to insulin action leads to an elevated blood sugar."[25]

In other words, anytime you eat simple carbohydrates your blood glucose level starts to rise immediately because the body begins turning it into glucose, which alerts the pancreas to release more insulin into the bloodstream.

Consuming additional simple carbohydrates will produce more glucose, which will call for yet more insulin. As each adds to its numbers in the bloodstream, the following is taking place: the traffic on your body's highways is increasing; your arteries are getting overcrowded with blood, insulin, glucose, fat, and waste material all fighting for space.

If triglyceride fats are also in the mix they may be narrowing some arteries by sticking to the walls and creating a bottleneck, backing up the ever increasing levels of insulin and glucose. That's the description of a clot. The end result is that fuel isn't going to get to some organs, possibly causing them to fail. If this happens in a critical artery supplying blood to the brain it could lead to a stroke.

The authors of *The Glucose Revolution* wrote, "Medical experts now believe that high glucose and insulin levels are one of the key factors responsible for heart disease and hypertension."[26]

So, the question is: if insulin is so important, what is it? If not provided from an external source, where in the body does it come from, and just what is its function?

To start, insulin is a hormone that is needed for cells to burn glucose, but strangely, it does not play an active part in the burning process. In fact, some say it's just a key that opens the cell's door to let glucose in.

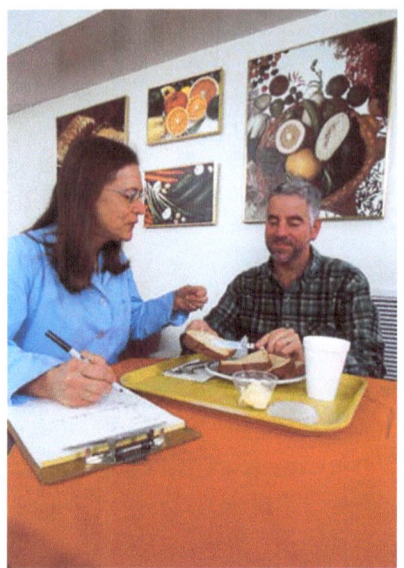

Considered from that point of view, if the cell door cannot be unlocked to let glucose in, carbohydrate metabolism cannot take place. Basically that's all there is to it. Insulin's primary function is to open the cell's door.

Image 12: Nutritionist Kay Behall works with study volunteer Dan Scholfield, who is consuming ultra-fine-ground bread in an experiment to evaluate its effect on blood glucose in insulin levels.

However, there is also a dark side to insulin: Author James Scala explains it this way: "If insulin only dealt with glucose metabolism, there would be no problem, but insulin does more. A secondary function of insulin is to help the kidneys retain sodium. In short, the excess insulin results in less sodium excretion (…) you know that this results in greater fluid retention." [27]

Let's digress for a moment. In Chapter 6, I had said the pancreas is the source of insulin. If the pancreas is so important, why don't we hear more about it?

Located behind the stomach, the pancreas is triggered to provide insulin whenever the digestive system senses a new supply of glucose or triglycerides. The pancreas is perhaps the most important gland of the digestive system since it also provides the enzymes for digesting proteins, carbohydrates, and all fats.

Additionally, in Chapter 3 (endnote 5) we had also been warned about letting an excess of simple carbohydrates show up in the bloodstream because it forces the pancreas to excrete surges of insulin.

Increases of both glucose and insulin in the bloodstream at the same time will show up as spikes in blood sugar levels. This is just another problem the body faces when insulin is released.

As vital a role as it plays in helping to supply the body's cells with fuel, insulin still looks like a major trouble maker for at least three reasons: It is directly responsible for getting diabetes under way, it indirectly causes high blood pressure, and it helps put and keep fat on our bodies.

Who needs enemies when we've got a friend like this? Unfortunately, we do. In fact, not only do we just need it, but our lives depend on it. So, let's get back to one of the problems it creates, namely diabetes. Just what is it?

In *Reversing Diabetes*, Dr. Julian Whitaker says, "Diabetes is a disorder of the body's means of utilizing glucose--a simple sugar that is the basic fuel that energizes our cells. When we talk about diabetes, we are generally referring to diabetes mellitus, sometimes called sugar diabetes."[28]

Dr. Whitaker continues his definition of diabetes by providing a general overview of the two types of this disorder:

TYPE 1 DIABETES, which used to be called juvenile diabetes, caused by a lack of insulin in the body, and always requires supplemental insulin, whereas:

TYPE 2 DIABETES (Diabetes Mellitus) usually, though not always, shows up in middle age or later. It does not reflect a lack of insulin but rather the inability of the body to use it effectively.

Remember, the pancreas is the only organ in the body that can produce insulin and once it wears out, the individual has to have insulin provided from an external source such as pills or by injection for the rest of his or her life.[29]

And, how often have we heard the following: "Too much fat (in the body) imposes stress on your heart, other organs, joints, and in many people causes high blood pressure."[30]

But, you argue—and rightly so because all of us have the same digestive process working on our food whether we're overweight or not—why do some people gain weight and see an increase in the waistline, but others don't?

There is a greater need for the overweight to recognize the danger they face because "fat" cell requires more insulin than the average cells does.

Author Scala explains why: "This doesn't mean that a person has more cells but that 'fat' cells simply can't efficiently or effectively use the insulin provided. The net outcome is that the body has to produce more insulin to compensate."[31]

Fortunately, "working the pancreas to death" can be reversed if the extra body weight is taken off early enough or is prevented from accumulating.

Remember this: Keeping the pancreas working overtime can wear out the gland so that insulin will eventually have to be provided from an external source, such as pills or injections.

Digressing again, the term "*fat*" cell needs an explanation.

Yes, there is such a thing as a "fat" cell. As a matter of fact, we were born with a fixed number of them. We've seen it all of our lives manifested as "baby fat" on infants and toddlers. They have a specific need for such cells because they store energy, provide insulation, and heat. They're ideal for the child because dietary fat can get into "fat" cells without the help of insulin.

In time, the amount of fat stored in "fat" cells will determine your weight and girth but their numbers will remain the same.

It has been suggested that the greatly overweight or obese, however, may be able to grow new ones because the ones they were born with can't hold any more fat.

Let's put it all together! Although we may diligently work to control what we eat by preparing modest portions of nutritious meals, most of our food will still be turned into sugar, a.k.a. glucose, which requires insulin to get into the body's cells.

But insulin is also used to help the kidneys hang on to sodium—the same sodium in the salt we've been told to avoid. Author Scala says, "And, we know that sodium, specifically salt, is a prime culprit in high blood pressure."[32]

In other words, what salt there is in our food is going to hang around longer because of the insulin. And, because water and sodium have an affinity for each other, more water is going to hang around, too, which makes our blood pressure go up. In other words, the heart has to work harder to flush the sodium, water, and waste products out of the kidneys.

On the other hand, the blood sugar level decreases because the concentration of glucose in the greater volume of retained water has been lowered.

Scala says, "The body is actually protecting itself from one evil, namely elevated blood sugar level (diabetes), by creating a lesser evil, high blood pressure. (hypertension)."[33]

It's obvious we can't eliminate our three silent killers, but we can control them by following the simple admonitions we've heard so often before:

Eat the right foods in moderation and exercise!

Chapter Eight

Prescription Medication

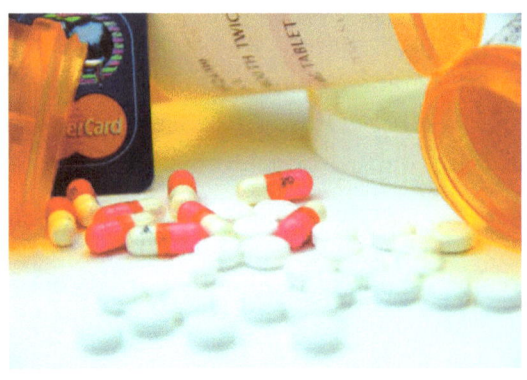

Image 13: When diet choices and health collide, the result can be expensive medications for the remainder of your life.

I hope this book has given you a chance to understand how these three debilitating diseases could be affecting your life as a result of eating excessive amounts of the "wrong" foods. You could reverse the trend by simply eating more of the "right" kind in smaller portions. To repeat the warning from Chapter 2—*Don't guess!* If you haven't visited your doctor recently, you might not know what your true medical condition is. Make that visit!

Your doctor will probably first address the problems that obesity poses and simply recommend eliminating or reducing fat, salt, and sugar in your diet; eating more of the "right" foods; and exercising.

If tests indicate that hypertension has also become a problem, your doctor will probably prescribe some medication for you to use while you follow a new diet and exercise protocol.

Now that we know something about the types of food we eat, how will the medicines prescribed for hypertension affect what you eat? As a matter of fact, they don't!

Let's backtrack and recall that the most serious of the three diseases is diabetes, which is a disorder that prevents the body from effectively using glucose, the end product of carbohydrates.

As I mentioned earlier, the disorder can be the result of overcrowded arterial freeways filled with insulin, glucose, and clot-producing triglyceride fat, which can stop the delivery of glucose to the cells completely.

The result can be fatal Dr. Julian Whitaker says: "If glucose is not removed from the bloodstream, the blood glucose level rises, and the diabetic condition results. If blood glucose elevates markedly (...) the blood becomes more acidic, a condition called diabetic ketoacidosis. A patient in this state may go into a diabetic coma and die."[34]

When insulin retains sodium, it also results in greater water retention, which, in turn, results in higher blood pressure. The purpose of some prescriptions is to remove excess water and salt from the kidneys.

Another obstacle to overcome is overcrowding of the arteries. Some prescriptions make the lining of the arteries more pliable, allowing them to increase in diameter. Still other medicines cause the heart to beat more forcefully, thus letting insulin and glucose get to their destination without getting hung up in "traffic."

Chapter Nine

Exercising

It's finally time to get off the couch and take on the other part of our doctor's recommendation to stop the onslaught of the three silent killers. It's time for us to exercise!

All of us know that exercising can burn off a few pounds but how does it prevent hypertension and more to the point, how can it stop diabetes? The best way to explain the benefits of exercise in this context is to refer to those authors already referenced throughout this book.

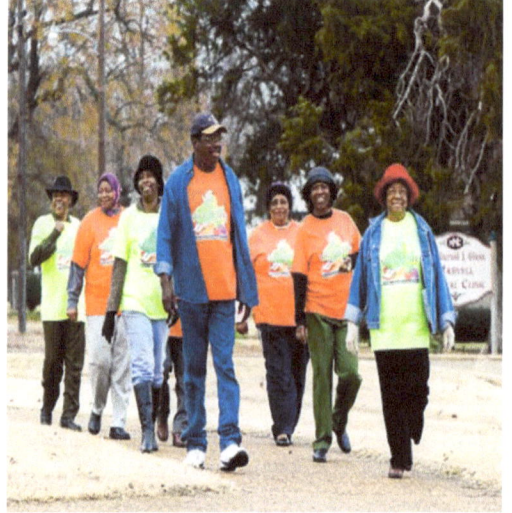

Image 14: Members of the Marvell Walking Club take a stroll on their community's recently refurbished walking trail (in Marvell, Arkansas).

Robert K. Cooper, author of *Low-Fat Living* offers some common-sense advice with the following: "If you just add a few active minutes here and there, you'll also be taking some giant strides toward controlling your dietary fat intake. Actions as simple as taking the stairs instead of the elevator or walking an extra block or two can help you neutralize natural cravings for high fat foods."[35]

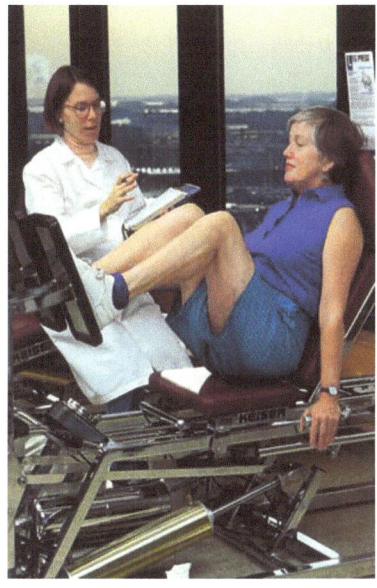

Image 15: The Human Nutrition Research Program is helping discover how people's nutritional needs differ by gender, age, activity level, and many other factors such as the impact of weight training on bones and calcium.

The authors of *The Glucose Revolution* emphasize the need for exercise with the following: "Exercise, or any physical activity, speeds up our metabolic rate. Exercise also makes our muscles better at using fat as a source of fuel. By improving the way insulin works, exercise increases the amount of fat we burn."[36]

Author Julian M. Whitaker of *Reversing Diabetes* says: "The glucose-reducing action of exercise was first demonstrated more than a hundred years ago, and a number of theories have been developed to explain how it works. One theory is that by dilating (opening) the blood vessels, exercise allows even small amounts of circulating insulin to be used, resulting in a fall of blood glucose. Another theory is that the exercising muscle might release some substance that acts like insulin and allows circulating glucose to enter the cells."[37]

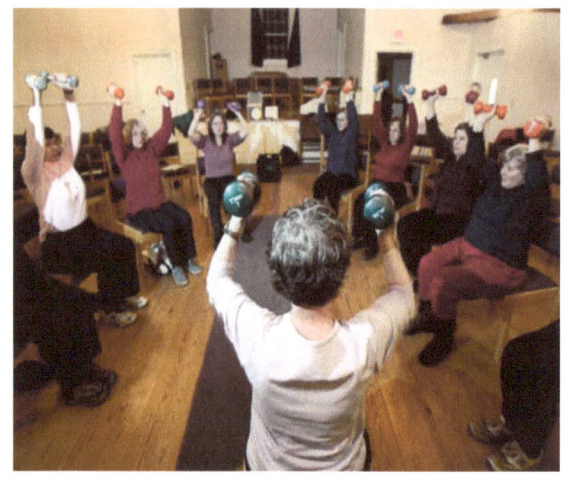

Image 16: Low impact exercise classes are available in most communities. Check with your doctor for suggestions of low impact and appropriate weight type exercise to maintain a healthy lifestyle.

Dr. Scala repeats the message: "Moderate regular exercise improves cardiac output, reduces blood pressure, and increases lean body mass... Improved cardiac output means the heart pumps more blood with each beat. In other words, regular exercise improves the pumping efficiency of the heart - it makes your heart a stronger muscle. ...after all, the heart is a muscle, and how do you improve the strength and flexibility of any muscle? Exercise, that's how! So, regular moderate exercise will improve the muscles being used in the exercise...including the heart."[38]

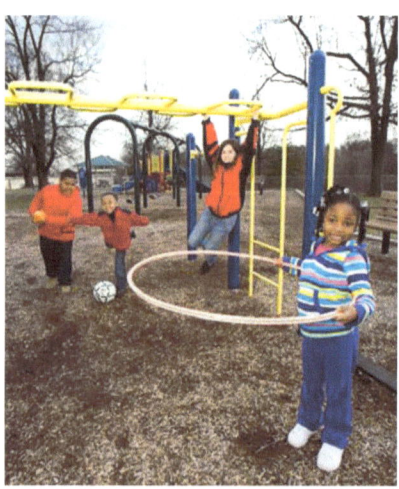

Do we really want obesity, hypertension, and diabetes controlling our lives? Naturally, the answer is **NO**! The choice has always been ours.

Image 17: Findings from Agricultural Research Service research may help kids enjoy becoming—and staying—physically active, a key to preventing childhood obesity. Less screen time, more play time.

My sincerest hope is that the simple explanations of how food affects you will motivate you to help yourself avoid the devastation any one of the three can bring you and those who love you. Once again, "The choice has always been yours."

Your body is yours to maintain. Your internal systems know best how to manipulate the foods they have to work with. Consequently, to the best of your ability, it's up to you to provide it with the proper materials it needs. My best wishes to you for a healthy rest of your life!!

Bob

References

Bass, Clarence. *"Shutdown Your Fat Genes – Turn on Your Thin Genes: The Fat Building Gene."* Clarence Bass' RIPPED Enterprises, http://www.cbass.com/FatGenes.htm.

Jennie Brand-Miller, Stephen Colagiuri, Kaye Foster-Powell and Thomas M.S. Wolever, *The Glucose Revolution: The Authoritative Guide to the Glycemic Index-The Groundbreaking Medical Discovery.*

Berkeley, CA: Marlowe & Company, 1999

Cooper, Robert K. *Low-Fat Living: Turn Off the Fat-Makers Turn On the Fat-Burners for Longevity Energy Weight Loss Freedom from Disease.* Emmaus PA: Rondale Press, Inc., 1996

Diabetes Fact Sheet. International Diabetes Institute, 2003, http://crlnsw. com.au/fileadmin/user_upload/National/ Sports_Trainers_Scheme/ HyperHighbloodglucoselevels.pdf

Editors of FC&A Publishing, Inc, ed. *Eat and Heal.* Peachtree City, GA: Frank Cawood and Associates, Inc, 2001.

"Flaxseeds". *The World's Healthiest Foods*. George Mateljan Foundation http://www.whfoods.com/genpage.php?tname=foodspice&dbid=81.

Kanade, Shrinivas. *"Triglycerides and Diabetes."* Buzzle.com: Intelligent Life on the Web. http://www.buzzle.com/articles/ triglycerides-and-diabetes.html.

Kiester, Edwin, and Sally Valente Kiester. *Eating Healthy Cookbook..* Des Moines, IA: Better Homes & Garden Books. 1986

Scala, James. *High Blood Pressure Relief Diet.* New York: NAL Penguin Inc. 1989

Whitaker, Julian M. *Reversing Diabetes.* New York: Warner Books, Inc. 1987

Wonderly, Kimberly. *"Do Carbohydrates Produce Triglycerides?"* Livestrong.com: The Limitless Potential of You. http://www.livestrong.com/article/432754-do-carbohydrates-produce-triglycerides.

Yeager, Selene. *Doctor's Book of Food Remedies: The Newest Discoveries in the Power of Food to Cure and Prevent Health Problems.* Emmaus, PA: Rodale Press, Inc. 1997

Endnotes

[1] Editors of FC&A Publishing, Inc., *Eat and Heal* (Peachtree City: Frank Cawood and Associates, Inc, 2001). 7

[2] *Gloria Rose, 200+ Recipes for Longer Life* Garden City Park, NY: Avery Publishing Group Inc, 1994). 23

[3] Jennie Brand-Miller, Stephen Colagiuri, Kaye Foster-Powell and Thomas M.S. Wolever, *The Glucose Revolution: The Authoritative Guide to the Glycemic Index—The Groundbreaking Medical Discovery* (Marlowe & Company, 1999). 10

[4] Selene Yeager, *Doctor's Book of Food Remedies: The Newest Discoveries in the Power of Food to Cure and Prevent Health Problems.* (Emmaus, PA: Rodale Press, Inc. 1997). 182

[5] Julian M Whitaker, *Reversing Diabetes* (New York: Warner Books, Inc. 1987). 119

[6] Ibid., 115

[7] Jennie Brand-Miller, Stephen Colagiuri, Kaye Foster-Powell and Thomas M.S. Wolever, *The Glucose Revolution: The Authoritative Guide*

to the Glycemic Index-The Groundbreaking Medical Discovery (Marlowe & Company, 1999). 42

[8] James Scala, *High Blood Pressure Relief Diet* (New York: NAL Penguin Inc. 1989). 116

[9] Ibid.

[10] Robert K Cooper, *Low-Fat Living: Turn Off the Fat-Makers Turn On the Fat-Burners for Longevity Energy Weight Loss Freedom from Disease* (Emmaus, PA: Rondale Press, Inc. 1996). 31

[11] Edwin Kiester and Sally Valente Kiester. *Eating Healthy Cookbook* (Des Moines, IA: Better Homes & Garden Books. 1986). 11

[12] Robert K Cooper, *Low-Fat Living: Turn Off the Fat-Makers Turn On the Fat-Burners for Longevity Energy Weight Loss Freedom from Disease.* (Emmaus, PA: Rondale Press, Inc. 1996). 31

[13] Selene Yeager,. *Doctor's Book of Food Remedies: The Newest Discoveries in the Power of Food to Cure and Prevent Health Problems* (Emmaus, PA: Rodale Press, Inc. 1997). 184

[14] Shrinivas Kanade, *"Triglycerides and Diabetes"* (Buzzle.com: Intelligent Life on the Web. 10 Jan. 2012) http://www.buzzle.com/articles/triglycerides-and-diabetes.html

[15] Kimberly Wonderly, *"Do Carbohydrates Produce Triglycerides?"* (Livestrong.com: The Limitless Potential of You. 10 Jan. 2012) <http://www.livestrong.com/article/432754-do-carbohydrates-produce-triglycerides>

[16] Shrinivas Kanade, *"Triglycerides and Diabetes"* (Buzzle.com: Intelligent Life on the Web. 10 Jan. 2012) <http://www.buzzle.com/articles/triglyc-erides-and-diabetes.html

[17] Selene Yeager, *Doctor's Book of Food Remedies: The Newest Discoveries in the Power of Food to Cure and Prevent Health Problems* (Emmaus, PA: Rodale Press, Inc. 1997). 184

[18] Robert K Cooper, *Low-Fat Living: Turn Off the Fat-Makers Turn On the Fat-Burners for Longevity Energy Weight Loss Freedom from Disease* (Emmaus, PA: Rondale Press, Inc. 1996). 33

[19] Selene Yeager, *Doctor's Book of Food Remedies: The Newest Discoveries in the Power of Food to Cure and Prevent Health Problems* (Emmaus, PA: Rodale Press, Inc. 1997). 184

[20] Clarence Bass, *"Shutdown Your Fat Genes – Turn on Your Thin Genes: The Fat Building Gene."* (Clarence Bass' RIPPED Enterprises. 10 Jan. 2012) <http://www.cbass.com/FatGenes.htm>

[21] *Diabetes Fact Sheet.* (International Diabetes Institute, 2003)

[22] Ibid.

[23] Editors of FC&A Publishing, Inc, ed., *Eat and Heal* (Peachtree City, GA: Frank Cawood and Associates, Inc. 2001). 162

[24] *"Flaxseeds," The World's Healthiest Foods* (George Mateljan Foundation. 10 Jan. 2012) http://www.whfoods.com/genpage.php?tname=foodspice&dbid=81>

[25] Gloria Rose, *200+ Recipes for Longer Life* (Garden City Park, NY: Avery Publishing Group Inc, 1994). 23

[26] Jennie Brand-Miller, Stephen Colagiuri, Kaye Foster-Powell and Thomas M.S. Wolever, *The Glucose Revolution: The Authoritative Guide to the Glycemic Index-The Groundbreaking Medical Discovery* (Marlowe & Company, 1999). 4

[27] James Scala, *High Blood Pressure Relief Diet* (New York: NAL Penguin Inc. 1989). 58

[28] Julian M Whitaker, *Reversing Diabetes* (New York: Warner Books, Inc. 1987). 5

[29] Ibid.

[30] Ibid., 254

[31] Ibid., 57

[32] Ibid., 27

[33] Ibid., 58

[34] Julian M Whitaker, *Reversing Diabetes* (New York: Warner Books, Inc. 1987). 6

[35] Robert K Cooper, *Low-Fat Living: Turn Off the Fat-Makers Turn On the Fat-Burners for Longevity Energy Weight Loss Freedom from Disease* (Emmaus, PA: Rondale Press, Inc. 1996). 102

[36] Jennie Brand-Miller, Stephen Colagiuri, Kaye Foster-Powell and Thomas M.S. Wolever, *The Glucose Revolution: The Authoritative Guide to the Glycemic Index-The Groundbreaking Medical Discovery* (Marlowe & Company, 1999). 65

[37] Julian M Whitaker, *Reversing Diabetes* (New York: Warner Books, Inc. 1987). 146

[38] James Scala, *High Blood Pressure Relief Diet* (New York: NAL Penguin Inc. 1989). 270

Images

1 Uppergi.gif. Public domain art. Work of the United States Federal Government under the terms of Title 17, Chapter 1, Section 105 of the US Code. 3. http://commons.wikimedia.org/wiki/File:Uppergi.gif

2 Digestive system with liver.png. Creative Commons Attribution-Share Alike 2.5 Generic. Author: Flynn, Gordon. 3.http://commons.wikimedia.org/wiki/File:Digestive_system_with_liver.png

3 d1829-43.jpg. USDA ARS Public domain art. http://www.ars.usda.gov/is/graphics/photos/jul10/d1829-43.htm Photo by Stephen Ausmus.

4 k8666-1.jpg. USDA ARS Public domain art. http://www.ars.usda.gov/is/graphics/photos/dec99/k8666-1.htm Fresh cut fruits and vegetables.

5 k7650-1.jpg. USDA ARS Public domain art. http://www.ars.usda.gov/is/graphics/photos/jun97/k7650-1.htm Photo by Scott Bauer.

6 d001-1.jpg. USDA ARS Public domain art. http://www.ars.usda.gov/is/graphics/photos/dec04/d001-1.htm

7 k9093-1.jpg. USDA ARS Public domain art. http://www.ars.usda.gov/is/graphics/photos/oct00/k9093-1.htm Photo by Peggy Greb.

8 k6027-8.jpg. USDA ARS Public domain art. http://www.ars.usda.gov/is/graphics/photos/mar98/k6027-8.htm Photo by Keith Weller.

9 k9988-1.jpg. USDA ARS Public domain art. 27 http://www.ars.usda.gov/is/graphics/photos/nov03/k9988-1.htm Photo by Stephen Ausmus.

10 d1529-1.jpg. USDA ARS Public domain art. http://www.ars.usda.gov/is/graphics/photos/oct09/d1529-1.htm

11 k9563-1.jpg. USDA ARS Public domain art. http://www.ars.usda.gov/is/graphics/photos/aug01/k9563-1.htm

12 k8870-1.jpg. USDA ARS Public domain art. http://www.ars.usda.gov/is/graphics/photos/may00/k8870-.htm

13 US_Army_52156_VA_warns_veterans_of_telephone_prescription_scam.jpg. http://commons.wikimedia.org/wiki/File:US_Army_52156_VA_warns_veterans_of_telephone_prescription_scam.jpg. 47 (public domain: US Army 52156 VA)

14 d429-18.jpg. USDA ARS Public domain art. http://www.ars.usda.gov/is/graphics/photos/mar06/d429-18.htm Photo by Stephen Ausmus.

15 k4610-12.jpg. USDA ARS Public domain art. http://www.ars.usda.gov/is/graphics/photos/nov03/k4610-12.htm

16 D067-25.jpg. USDA ARS Public domain art. http://www.ars.usda.gov/is/graphics/photos/may05/D067-25.htm

17 d1723-1.jpg. USDA ARS Public domain art. http://www.ars.usda.gov/is/graphics/photos/mar10/d1723-1.htm

About the Author

I was born in Shanghai, China, a very multicultural and cosmopolitan city in 1926, and where I spent my entire childhood from the beginning of the Sino-Japanese War in 1937 till the end of World War 2 in 1945.

After the outbreak of World War 2, along with a thousand American, Britons and other allied civilians I was interned in the Chapei Civilian Assembly Center one of several camps located in Shanghai. From February 1943 to the end of the war in August 1945, my two and a half years as a civilian prisoner of war gave me a unique opportunity to experience the effects of some food deprivation and observe its result on the interned population.

Thankfully, the administrators of the camp provided an adequate amount of food to keep us alive. By default we became vegans since meat and fish products were not available. I don't recall eating fish during that time because the waters around the city were extremely polluted. Consequently, only baskets of vegetables were brought in every day or two while bags of rice were maintained at a constant level.

In researching the material for this booklet, I can appreciate a fortuitous situation that took place at the time. When we were interned, some materials were of no use to the Japanese. With that in mind, they transported books to the camp from the American and English schools as well as several tons of cracked wheat. It may seem strange that they would have given us a valuable item such as wheat. Sent by the American Red Cross for Chinese refugees before World War 2, cracked wheat was not a dietary staple of either the Chinese or the Japanese at the time. Whether we liked it or not we had a chance to have cracked wheat for breakfast for two and a half years without anything like milk or sugar to flavor it.

Looking back over the years, my recollection is that out of the population of a thousand, only two internees died—both of cancer. I think that was remarkable considering the limited medical facilities available and the number of potential diseases that could have killed us.

I must have forgotten my early experiences, because recent physical exams diagnosed me as "obese"—not just fat. Tests showed that I also had high blood pressure and was pre-diabetic. Thankfully, my medical doctor provided instructions and recommendations that caused me to lose weight. In addition, she had also prescribed medications that brought my blood pressure numbers down into the "normal" range. Overall the general admonition was to eat less and exercise more.

Editor's note:

At the conclusion of World War 2, Mr. Hegamin finally arrived in the U.S. November, 1945. He served in the U.S. Air Force (1948-52) during the Korean War, assigned to Goose Bay, Labrador, and one of its detachments in the Arctic, concluding his enlistment in the Mojave Desert.

He completed his pre-engineering at Columbia University and graduated from Seattle University in 1966 with Bachelor of Science degrees in Electrical Engineering and General Science.

His list of civic involvement and activism are highlighted by his service as a member on the Washington State Board for Community College Education (1977 - 1979) and the King County Personnel Board (1990 - 1994).

Mr. Hegamin worked for the Boeing Company in Seattle and retired as an electrical engineer from Seattle City Light in 1988.

www.ingramcontent.com/pod-product-compliance
Lightning Source LLC
Chambersburg PA
CBHW050817290526
45792CB00001B/154